How to Overcome Anxiety and Depression

Roadmap to Living Above Fears, Worries, and Anxiety.

ADEGBOYE Samuel

TABLE OF CONTENTS

Introduction

Depression is more being unhappy or feeling sad. Once in a while, you can feel unmotivated, low, angry, or upset. But melancholy is more than just being down.

Sometimes we ask ourselves a series of questions such as can I get out of the state? The battle continues until you find yourself doing nastic things because of worries. One of the greatest things to deal with to live out of fears is your mind.

Depression is a disorder – a mood disorder that affects how an individual behaves feels, thinks, reacts, interacts in a long time (continuous reoccurrence of this disorder for a minimum of two weeks show you are depressed).

The symptoms of this disorder can range from fatigue and hopelessness to physical pain, loss of interest in Life, or suicidal thoughts. In the diagnostic and statistical manual (DSM-5), it was stated that when a person sees these symptoms or signs continuously within the same two weeks or more, he or she is experiencing a depressive disorder.

When you discover you are suffering from depression, the next step is how you can go about it.

Chapter one

What does it mean to be depressed?

Depression has taken over the lives of individuals and teenagers in the world. However, it is irrespective of race, countries, continent, tribe, region, community, or society you find yourself. One way or the other, you find yourself depressed with one or more things.

Sometimes people call it mood swing – a rapid and extreme change in mood from excessively *happiness* to desperately *Miserable.* It is a general meaning given to mood swing, yea! It is correct. But sometimes a swing in your mood can cause you to go into a deep reflection that can provide a solution to a problem. However, how often does that happen? Some say of Mood Disorder – an affective disorder. But whichsoever ways, you can be happy now and within a twinkle of an eye, swing to a saddened mood.

We are on the planet where we can't tell what can happen to us in the next hour. Well, an hour maybe extreme to consider. Let me say in the next second. Being alive at this moment does not guarantee your existence the next second. Being healed this moment from a particular sickness does not ensure it won't reoccur in the next second. Being healthy this time doesn't mean you won't break down in the next second. Being accepted in a particular niche or environ doesn't give you complete assurance that you won't be neglected and abandoned in a moment. Living a peaceful life does not mean war won't break-in in a second.

Views on Depression

Most times, we puzzle ourselves with the history of depression to be able to get over our worries. We read a lot of books, magazines, journals, and encyclopedia to understand how we came about depression. And gradually, despair grows into the significant sickness we fight with day in and out. Some medical practitioners have deviated a little from their profession to be able to get a solution to this disease that outbroke itself to become the world's most known issues. Records show that people who commit suicide daily as increased geometrically in most countries, and the root problem is *Depression.* Okay, my dear friend, let look into it together; what do you think will make a rich man wakes up a day and take some poisons to end up in the grave? You won't have known the secret thing he or she must have been battling with over time. But you will later discover that he was depressed.

While no individual is credited with the discovery of depression, there are a whole set of great leaders that have led --and continue to donate --to our developing understanding of precisely what this illness is. To be able to understand the way investigators, physicians, and psychologists consider this condition nowadays, it will be helpful to look back on the history of depression.

Depression in Early Age

One of the most initial discoveries of what is now known as depression appeared in Mesopotamia in the second millennium B.C. In this account, depression was seen as a spiritual issue rather than a physical. Similar to other mental illnesses, it was believed to be caused by demonic activities. As such, the priests were seen to be the proper agents that treat the problem rather than the physicians. This ideology grew in diverse cultures like Romans, ancient greeks Chinese, Egyptians, and Babylonians, and cause people to believe demons and evil spirits cause depression. Therefore, it was often dealt with by methods such as physical restraint, beatings, starvation in an attempt to drive out the demons.

Hippocrate's view on Depression

As far as little significance was placed on physical causes, Hippocrates – a Greek physician is credited with the belief that depression was caused by an imbalance in four body fluids of the body system, which includes humour: black bile, yellow bile, phlegm, and blood. He specifically said depression was a result of an excess of black bile in the spleen. And his treatment of depression includes; exercise, bloodletting, baths, and diet.

Cicero's view on Depression

In contrast to Hippocrates' ideology, Cicero, who was a philosopher, said depression is a psychological issue. It results from mental effects such as Rage, Fear, and Grieve. Before the common era, in spite of propositions by some physicians and philosophers to believe that depression is more of a mental and physical cause, most people, especially educated Romans still believe that depression and psychological illness is caused by demons or God's wrath.

Depression in 18th and 19th century

During the 18th and 19th centuries, which was also called the Age of Enlightenment, depression was seen as a weakness in temperament, which is inherited and cannot be changed. It was said that people with the condition should be locked up or shunned. Toward the latter part of the Age of Enlightenment, doctors began to suggest the idea that aggression was at the root of this condition. Other doctors spoke of depression as resulting from internal conflicts between what you want and what you know is right. And yet others sought to identify the physical causes of this condition.

From my discovery, depression can be psychological, physical, or spiritual. Whichever way, what matters here is to discover the root of what depresses you and tackle it.

If mental, how do I treat it? If physical, how do I treat it? If spiritual, how do I treat it? We seek to find answers to all these questions, to be able to handle our type of depression. This book will be discussing depression as more of a physical and mental illness.

Chapter two
DEPRESSION AND SADNESS?

One of the questions you must ask yourself is, does being sad also mean being depressed? Knowing that the primary symptom associated with depression is sadness, it can be challenging to understand how to make a clear difference between the two mental states.

But base on the factors that surround depression, it is more than just feeling sad, and not only by a measure of degree. The difference between these two psychological states is not based on the degree to which an individual is not active but somewhat in

- a combination of factors relating to the duration of these negative feelings.
- Bodily impact.
- The effect upon the person's ability to function in daily life.

- And Other symptoms.

Facts about Sadness that differentiate it from Depression

1. Sadness is a normal emotion that every person will experience at some point in his or her life. It may be as a result of;

   - Job loss,

   - When a relationship ends,

   - or the death of a loved one,

   Sadness is typically caused by some particular situation, event, or person.

   During the depression, however, no such trigger is needed. A depressed person feels hopeless or sad about everything that surrounds him or her. This individual may have every reason in the world to be happy, and yet they lose the ability to experience joy or pleasure over everything.

2. In sadness, you might feel remorse for something you said or did, but you won't experience any permanent sense of guilt or worthlessness as with depression. One of the symptoms of depression is this kind of negative thought patterns and self-diminishing sign.

3. With sadness, you might feel down for a day or two, but you are still able to enjoy things like food, games, your favourite TV show, or spending time with friends and family. But for a person suffering from depression, activities that they once enjoyed are no longer pleasurable to them.

4. When you experience sadness triggered by a particular situation or event, you are still able to sleep as you usually would, remain elevated to perform your daily

activities, and maintain your attitude to food while depression is associated with severe disruption of sleeping patterns and usual eating habits, and not wanting to get out of bed all day.

5. Finally, non-depressive sadness does not cause self-suicidal inclinations and self-harm. Those struggling with severe depression may have thoughts of death, or suicide, self-harm, or have a suicide plan.

How do I know I am depressed?

The following lists are symptoms that can help you know that you are experiencing a depressive disorder. Once you begin to notice at least five or more of these symptoms within the same two weeks, you need to get a solution in how to get out of this state.

1. When you discover yourself in a depressed mood most times and daily.

2. When you notice that you have diminished interest or pleasure in all activities, or almost all, activities most times of the day, and mostly every day.

3. When you begin to notice tangible weight loss when not dieting, or decrease in appetite mostly every day.

4. When you begin to notice that your thought slows down and physical movement reduces in rate, this observation may be from people around you.

5. When you mostly feel a loss of energy or fatigue daily.

6. When you discover you feel inappropriate guilt or worthlessness most time every day, start working towards treating depression.

7. When you start feeling a reduced ability to concentrate or think, most of the time, daily.

8. When you begin to have repeated thoughts of suicidal ideation or death, without a specific plan.

9. When you start reacting aggressively or angrily to each of your necessities.

Chapter three
Myth about depression

The reality of "death by suicide" universally takes the core stage than it is being addressed. Presently, the world is admitting the implications of untreated depression. The account of people who died by committing suicide reveals that four (4) out of six victims have symptoms of major depression. If depression is fought against, some educative sessions will be taken to enlighten a lot of individual on debunking myths. Some of these untreated depression result from this inherent belief of these myths. It won't be funny when you, family, friends, relatives or colleagues suffer from this illness, and you can't decipher between facts and fictions that surround the ailment to overcome it.

The earlier you get to limelight on what depression is all about and break out from the myths that surround it, the closer are you to its complete cure. The earlier we eradicate the myths behind depression, the earlier it will be understood by the masses.

The following are ten (10) myths about depression that has become the general knowledge of masses.

1. ***Depression is another word for sadness:*** Since this has been earlier discussed, I will not dwell much on it. But this is becoming generally accepted myths, even among the educated ones. When you are sad, it doesn't mean you are depressed. Sadness is a symptom of depression while ***it is NOT depression.*** Sadness is a temporary experience, and it is triggered

by an event. For example,you can be sad as a result of your sophisticated phone damage, but sooner you will get over it. In the course of the moment of your sadness, if eventually, you have been expecting a higher version of that your phone, and it was sent at that instance, the grief would be eradicated immediately. Note that sadness is just one of the negative symptoms that accompany depression, but it is not depression.

2. ***When you are being told you have depression because you are mentally weak***: Most times, people term patient that is suffering from depression, mentally weak person. Are they right? NO. But in that sense,they may be right. Not all people who are mentally weak are depressed, but when you are depressed, your psychological health will grow weak.

3. ***The only cause of depression is a traumatic event:***

Sometimes we carry this mind, depression only happens when a traumatic incident occurs to someone. It has been proven that it doesn't happen in all cases. However, trauma is one of the primary factors that trigger depression, but sometimes some persons get over shock soon and continue living their lives. There are some cases where change of environment,leaving your family to another location can cause depression. These are not traumatic incidents. We must not confine ourselves to this myth that depression is caused only by traumatic events. It won't help notice or help those suffering from it without record of any terrible incident happening to them.

4. *It is not real illness; it is just depression:* This is another myth that has endanger a lot of persons suffering from depression. Most people do not see

depression as a big problem. They casualise it until the victim gets to the point of committing suicide. This is strict attention we must look into; depression is a real illness and needs a special treatment.

5. *Oh, it is just in your head:* Our perceptions about things are different. But the wrong impression can burn down a whole mansion without leaving a pin. Depression is a head thing – while the source is from the brain, the effect spread to all other parts of the body in a short time. The way depression affects people is different because of our differences.

6. *Depression is not for Real men:* Waoh! This is one of the trending myth. Real men do not get depressed. And it has made a lot of men hide till death. Statistically, women are prone to depression when compared to men. But that doesn't mean men don't suffer from depression. The world term Real men to

those that are rugged in their deals, they can fight through any path, they are active and energetic, and we believe this kind of people don't suffer depression. Do you know what happens to this kind of men? Because of how the world sees them. They hide when depressed it grows worst beyond control. The myth makes it difficult for men to open up. To reduce the rate at which people die of depression, we must educate everyone against this myth.

7. ***When you talk about depression, it grows worst:*** When depressed, share your story. It helps reduce the intensity of it implications.we have been made to believe that when you discuss your problems to people, they add to them rather than finding a solution to them. But in a good sense, when you present your depressed state to people, you will be able to know how to go about it and who is causing more problem

for you.

8. ***When you are depressed, all you need is an anti-depressant:*** It partially true, but not exact. There are different therapies, used to treat depression, which anti-depressant is one of it. Most people believe the answer to depression is to get an anti-depressant for the patient. No! Doctor prescribe medications base on how the state of depression has grown and even add other therapies for better improvement.

9. ***If you are depressed, you will not be happy again:*** Those that are depressed also have happy moments. Being depressed doesn't mean you will never be comfortable or happy all through that moment; it doesn't mean you are 100% depressed of all the time. Remember that some people are excellent when it comes to hiding their feelings, you will always see them smiling, and they can make sure you don't shift

the mood. But right inside they are battling with depression. This is a myth; being depressed does not mean you won't have happy moments.

10. ***When you are depressed, you are miserable:*** This is a bit harsh. When you are depressed, it does not mean you are miserable or worthless. You are not in that state of worthlessness. Depression is an illness, and it is bound to leave you when it is appropriately managed. Do not encourage people with this myth; it can go as long as destroying an individual all through his life on earth.

Although, there are still some myths, but these are a common myth that has eaten the mind of people up on depression, and the implications have grown worst. When we educate ourselves against these myths, we would have a reduced rate at which people commit suicide because of depression.

Chapter four
TYPE OF DEPRESSION

There are many different types of depression, which will be mentioned below. Some of these types are caused by events or occurrences of life, and others by chemical changes in the brain. As this study continues, you will notice some symptoms of depressive disorder in some types overlap, but you must understand that there are fundamental differences.

Understanding the types of depression will streamline our focus on a question everyone should ask him/herself. *What kind of depression do I have?* When you take some time to understand the different types, it can help to start a journey to diagnose and recover from the form. Also, it will significantly help you when you talk to any mental health practitioner or doctor, and it will aid the doctor in getting the right depression diagnosis that you need.

Psychotic Depression

A study from the National Alliance on Mental Illness shows that twenty percent of patients suffering from depression have grown so severe into psychotic problems. It is a study that was thoroughly taken to discover the result of depressive disorder in people. When a patient is diagnosed with major depressive disorder with psychotic symptoms, he or she is said to be suffering from both the combination of the symptoms of psychosis and depression − a psychological state of disorganised behaviour and thoughts, delusions, or hallucinations.

Early signs of psychosis

These are signs seen when a person begins to lose contact with reality. When you start to notice the following signs in an individual, you need to be more cautious. The following are the symptoms of psychosis.

- The person starts withdrawing socially.

- He or she starts developing intense and inappropriate emotions.

- Extreme obsession.

- A rapid decline in personal hygiene.

- A consistent drop in performance level in school or at work.

How to diagnose Psychotic depression?

Psychotic depression can be characterised by an individual experiencing Major depressive disorder with psychotic symptoms. A patient with psychotic depression will be diagnosed if the symptoms have lasted for two weeks on more, and he or she is experiencing hallucinations or delusions. There are two types of psychotic depression, and both have features of illusion and delusion.

1. Major depressive disorder with Mood-congruent psychotic features: in this situation, the individual is suffering from the major depressive disorder with

Mood-congruent symptoms. That is, the picture of delusions and hallucinations is what makes the individual depressed.

2. Major depressive disorder with Mood-incongruent psychotic features: in this situation, the individual is suffering from the major depressive disorder with Mood-incongruent symptoms. That is, the picture of delusions and hallucinations is not in what makes the individual depressed.

Psychotic depression and schizophrenia

Can we conclude that psychotic depression and schizophrenia are the same? How do we define depression? It is a mood disorder, and psychotic depression can be summarised to be a mood disorder with psychotic features. However, schizophrenia is a psychological illness. Despite that, both terms psychosis symptoms in common. That doesn't mean psychotic depression will develop into schizophrenia. But schizophrenia patients can be depressed because of the condition that surrounds the illness.

Major depression
Major depressive disorder, as it is known, can also be called clinical or Unipolar depression. It happens when someone has a persistent feeling of sadness, a lack of interest in outdoor activities, or any of the symptoms that will be mentioned below within two weeks. The following symptoms characterise the major depressive disorder. When you have at least five or more of these symptoms continuously for two or more weeks, you are experiencing major depression.

- When you lose interest or pleasure in your activities.

- You are feeling of agitation or restlessness.

- Unfocus.

- Aggressive reactions to loved ones.

- Irritability.

- You are isolating yourself from people around you.

- The consciousness of guilt or guilt

- Pessimistic in thoughts.

- Regular sleeping habits.

- Exhaustion and lethargy.

- Suicidal thoughts.

- Weight loss

Can Major Depression be cured?

Major depression is a disorder that can live with an individual all through his or her life if it is not managed correctly. In regards to some of the symptoms of major depressive disorder, it is considered not curable. But beyond this view, there is no depression that is not curable when you get the right treatment.

For major depression disorder, it can be managed if it is tackled with the right treatment.

What are treatments available for Major Depression?

After some studies, the following treatments were discovered for the management of major depressive disorder;

- Cognitive Behaviour Therapy (CBT).

- Psychotherapy.

- Anti-depressant medications.

- Natural Treatment.

- Electroconvulsive therapy (ECT).

Any of the treatments can be used depending on individuality differences. But the best treatment for this disorder is the combination of medication and therapy.

Atypical depression

Similar to major depression, but with other symptoms such as feeling extremely weak, eating more than usual, sleeping for excessive amounts of time, and putting on weight, and feeling extremely sensitive to being rejected by others. It may be one of the most pronounced types of depression. Atypical depression is not the usual persistent hopelessness or sadness that made up significant types of depression.

Symptoms of atypical depression

- Overeating.

- Irritability.

- Sensitivity to rejection.

- Oversleeping.

- Heaviness in arms and legs.

- Quick reaction to relationship problems.

- Emotional instability.

One of the exciting parts of a person suffering from atypical depression is the ability to improve after a positive event

The severity of atypical depression

Atypical depression is a severe mental health condition, and it has a high risk of anxiety disorder and suicide thought. Teens and teenagers, students, young adults are prone to have this type of depression. It occurs in the early years of an individual and can stay a long time in them. This type of depression must be attended to as soon as possible to stop its action and effect that may lead to suicidal thoughts or even death.

Can atypical depression be cured?

From practitioners, there is no typical treatment that can cure atypical depression. But it is believed that the combination of both psychotherapy and medications, it can successfully be managed. Someone suffering from this type of depression can be encouraged to always stay in a pleasant and happy environment. He/ she must be prevented from staying alone because loneliness may trigger its effect.

Possible treatment for atypical depression.

As it was said above, it is advisable to use both medications and psycho treatment for atypical depression. Some possible treatments include; monoamine oxidase inhibitors and tricyclic antidepressants, which are the most common medication prescribed for the treatment of atypical depression.

Persistent depressive disorder (Dysthymia)

This depression disorder is also called Dysthymia. This type of depression that lasts for years and interfere with daily life, relationship, and work. Dysthymia is a long term type of depression. It makes an individual find it difficult to be happy even in a pleasant and joyous environment. The symptoms of a person suffering from dysthymia include; gloomy, complaining, and pessimistic nature.

Nature develops over time as the disorder continues. Symptoms of dysthymia appear and disappear but generally don't disappear for more than two months. The intensity of the symptoms can also change as time goes.

Comparing persistent and Major Depression Disorder

The kind of depressed mood a person suffering from dysthymia (persistent depressive disorder) experience is not as severe as a major depressive disorder. But both depressions share some common symptoms like Loss of pleasure, feelings of sadness, and hopelessness. For someone to be diagnosed with major depressive disorder, the symptoms must be present for two weeks. But for dysthymia, the patient must have been suffering from the symptoms for two or more years.

High-functioning depression and dysthymia

High-functioning depression is a term used for those suffering from dysthymia or persistent depressive disorder because of the severe nature of this type of depression. People suffering from this type of depression continue to live life robotically. They appear beautiful to those around them, but they die inside.

Double depression

Double depression occurs when people suffering from dysthymia begin to have worse symptoms that can lead to the full syndrome of Major depressive disorder with their formal dysthymia. It is called double depression because the patient continues to manage both major depression and dysthymia.

Bipolar Depressive Disorder

Bipolar disorder is also called manic depression. Bipolar depression is a mental health illness that causes extreme disorderliness of mood, behaviour, thought, the period of sleep, and energy. Manic depression does not just create "feeling down" it leads to a state of having suicidal thoughts and later builds up to a feeling of endless energy and euphoria. This swing of mood can occur a couple of times every week or sporadically show up just two times in a year.

Some treatments can be given to an individual suffering from bipolar depression, such as Mood stabilisers – it is used to regulate mood swings that come with bipolar disorder. An example of mood stabiliser is lithium. Some other prescription can be used, such may include medications like antipsychotics and antidepressants.

Can Bipolar disorder be cured?

Bipolar disorder can be successfully managed by combining psychotherapy and medications. It is advisable to treat any depression that can lead to bipolar disorder. So far, studies are still in progress on how to cure bipolar depression. It will be better to prevent it than trying to cure it.

Is bipolar disorder Genetic?

Since scientists have not been able to give the right conclusion on, maybe bipolar disorder is genetic but has been able to gather 60 – 80 % facts on its innate nature. They were able to discover that hereditary plays a large percentage when it comes to having bipolar disorder. It means the first possibility for a person to have this type of disease is to know may be any of your relatives have once suffered the sickness.

What are the differences between bipolar one (1) and bipolar two (2) disorder?

Since all types of bipolar depressive disorder have extraordinarily high or low symptoms, bipolar one (1) disorder and bipolar two (2) disorder have their unique differences. The significant difference between the two diseases is the severity of the manic features.

For bipolar one (1), the individual suffers from manic symptoms – also known as elevated mood. The sign is highly severe when compared with bipolar two (2).

While for bipolar two (2) disorder, the individual suffers from hypomania symptom – a less severe form of mania that results in behaviours that are peculiar to that individual but irrational to the society at large.

Premenstrual depression (Premenstrual Dysphoric Disorder)

When a woman feels extremely unhappy just before her monthly period, and the symptoms go away after her period starts (also called premenstrual dysphoric disorder).

Premenstrual depression is known as ***Premenstrual Dysphoric Disorder (PMDD)***. It is a mood disorder that is hormone-based, cyclic, and considered a disabling and severe form of premenstrual syndrome. According to the study and research in the American Journal of Psychiatry,

5% of women are diagnosed with Premenstrual Dysphoric Disorder (PMDD), while 85% of women experience premenstrual syndrome (PMS).

The following core symptoms show you are suffering from premenstrual dysphoric disorder (PMDD); anxiety, depressed mood, physical and behavioural aggression.

For proper treatment on PMDD, a woman must have experienced these symptoms for a year or more continuously during her menstrual cycle.

Differences Between Premenstrual Dysphoric Disorder (PMDD) and Premenstrual Syndrome (PMS)

PMDD is a more severe condition than PMS. In the days leading and during women's menstrual period, it is usual for women to have mood fluctuation. Anxiety, suicidal thoughts, and psychological symptoms of depression do not occur with premenstrual syndrome. The symptoms present with PMS do not generally interfere with daily activities and are less severe in their effect.

Medications for Premenstrual Dysphoric Disorder

There are medications approved by the FDA to help alleviate the symptoms of premenstrual Dysphoric Disorder (PMDD). For the treatment of symptoms of PMDD related to anxiety and mood, the following medications can be used.

- Selective serotonin reuptake inhibitors (SSRIs); it is a group of antidepressant.

- Fluoxetine.

- Sertraline.

- Paroxetine hydrochloride.

The medications mentioned above has been approved by the Food and Drug Administration (FDA).

How long does Premenstrual Dysphoric

Disorder Last?

Women observe their menstrual cycle every month. Therefore the symptoms of PMDD occur each month before and during menstruation. The symptoms of PMDD begin 5 to 10 days before menstruation and decrease in severity during the menstruation as you approach the end of the menstrual cycle for each month. After the cycle, the symptoms stop until the next menstrual period. Since this cycle is part of women's nature, the tendency of PMDD occurring is high. For a lady that just started menstruation, she experiences premenstrual dysphoric Disorder, but as time goes on, she can manage it to overcome it.

If not properly treated, a woman can nurse this form of depression for as long as she still experiences a menstrual cycle.

Seasonal patterns of depression

When a person only gets symptoms of depression each winter and autumns and feels better each spring and summer, sometimes called *'seasonal affective disorder.'* Symptoms are usually mild (e.g., overeating, sleeping too much, having trouble getting up in the morning, tiredness during the day, and putting on weight).

The seasonal affective disorder is a depression that occurs as a result of a change in season. Anybody who suffers from this type of depression notices symptoms during the same period every year. For example, the symptoms may also occur during winter or summer or autumn of every year. Whichsoever, the symptoms can start mild and increase to be more severe as the weeks go on. For some persons, symptoms can begin during the fall and continue during the winter. SAD can also occur during summer or spring. Symptoms of depression may include fatigue, loss of interest and pleasure in activities, and hopelessness. Individuals who experience SAD in winter have the following symptoms;

- Frequent oversleeping.

- Relationships problem.

- Craving for carbohydrate gain.

- Heaviness in legs and arms.

Cause of Seasonal Affection Disorder (SAD)

Psychologists and experts have worked as much to suggest the causes of SAD. But the exact reason is still not apparent. There have been some hypothesis related to the root of seasonal affective disorder at the onset, and they include;

- Physical illness.

- Traumatic life event.

- High melatonin levels.

- Low serotonin levels.

Can a seasonal pattern of depression happen in summer?

This type of depression is more common during this period – summer more than you can imagine. More than 10% of those suffering from seasonal affective disorder start noticing the sign during summer months. This shows that seasonal patterns of depression can happen in summer.

How can the seasonal affective disorder be treated?

The following range of treatment can be given to an individual suffering from Seasonal Affection Disorder (SAD);

- Psychotherapy.

- Medications.

- Light Therapy.

- Combinations of light therapy, psychotherapy, and medications.

- Talk therapy will be of good use for a SAD patient. For example, a psychotherapist can discover abnormalities in thoughts and behaviours that cause depression. Therefore teach positive ways of managing the symptoms.

Situational Depression

Situational depression is also known as adjustment disorder or reactive depression. It is a depression experienced in a short period when stressed. It occurs as a result of stress from work or other related activities. This kind of grief is hinged to a change that may arise unexpectedly in our everyday life. Example of events that cause situational depression include;

- Loss of friend (s) or Family member.

- Loss of Job.

- Divorce.

- Illness.

- Relationship Problem.

These are unexpected events that an individual would not have thought but suddenly arises. It is called adjustment disorder because of the person's readjustment to balance his or her everyday life after the experience.

Often, the symptoms start ninety days after the event.

Diagnosis of situational depression

For a person to be diagnosed with situational depression, he or she must have been experiencing behavioural or psychological symptoms three months after an identifiable stressor or event that is beyond normal response. The signs will continue for a long time and later develop into major depressive disorder if not treated.

The uniqueness of situational depression

An individual suffering from situational depression is likely to be experiencing all the symptoms associated with major depressive disorder. What makes situational depression difference from others is that it is a short-term occurrence that happens as a result of an unexpected event. Situational depression stops when an individual can adapt to the changes before him. It is not like a major depressive disorder that is seen as a result of chemical imbalances in the brain.

Prenatal and postnatal depression (peripartum or postpartum depression)

During pregnancy, when a woman has symptoms of depression or after giving birth (also called perinatal depression or peripartum depression or Postpartum depression).

The crying bouts and sad feelings that follow childbirth are known as the Baby blues. This feeling of sadness after birth is associated with the hormonal changes that occur in the body system. Baby blues tend to reduce one or two weeks after delivery. There are some women (although one in seven) that experiences deep depression beyond baby blues. However, when a woman struggles with worry, anxiety, or sadness for several weeks or more after childbirth, she may be experiencing Postpartum depression (PPD). Some of the symptoms or signs you will see to know you are suffering from peripartum or postpartum depression includes;

- Having feelings of anger and irritation.

- You are having feelings of tiredness most of the day.

- Changes occur in sleeping and eating habits.

- Sudden loss of interest in activities, including sex.

- You are feeling depressed and inactive for several weeks or more.

- A sudden withdrawal from friends and family.

- Anxiety, worry, racing thoughts, or panic attacks.

Why does peripartum or postpartum depression occur?

The study shows that the exact cause of this type of depression is unknown. But it is thought to be a result of some factors including; the physical changes that occur as a result of pregnancy worry about parenthood, the fright of travail, the pain of delivery, some times when a pregnancy or distribution is complicated. During pregnancy, some unfavourable factors that may include restriction to do their usual activities can also be the cause of PPD.

When does postpartum depression start?

Postpartum depression may not start immediately after childbirth. Sometimes the symptoms may begin a few weeks or months after child delivery. It may be during the first year of the baby.

Women who suffer from PPD may tend to have the worst depression, such as major depression afterward.

Disruptive Mood Dysregulation disorder – DMDD

This type of depressive disorder was discovered in recent times. It appeared in the DSM-5 in 2013. DSM is a diagnostic and statistical Manual of Mental Disorder. In this manual, Disruptive Mood Dysregulation Disorder was classified as a type of depressive disorder. Children who suffer from DMDD find it challenging to regulate their emotions and moods properly. As a result of this, they frequently respond verbally or behaviourally with a temper outburst during frustration. During this outburst, feel persistent and chronic irritation.

Can children overcome DMDD?

When you discover that your child has DMDD, seek the indulgence of a mental health professional for right counsel. Children may not be able to properly manage DMDD without learning how to regulate their moods and emotions. As parents, take the extra mile to visit a mental health practitioner for proper procedures.

Treatment for Disruptive Mood Dysregulation disorder – DMDD

To treat DMDD, we must use the combination of parent management skills and psychotherapy. This is the first step to take on how to educate children on how to control their moods and emotions. However, if this method is not sufficient for your child, you can use medications.

Difference between Bipolar disorder and Disruptive Mood Dysregulation disorder – DMDD

The significant symptom of DMDD is irritation, while the primary symptom of bipolar disorder is a manic or hypomanic trend. Although both depressions can cause irritability, DMDD irritable mood is chronic and severe, while bipolar depression irritable mood tends to occur sporadically.

Some other forms of depression

These different forms of depression either have a relationship with the type of depression listed above or are the other types of it.

Clinical depression

Depression that's been diagnosed by a professional. This is not a type of depression – it could include any kind.

Unipolar depression

The opposite of bipolar depression. Unipolar depression includes any depression when a person doesn't have bipolar disorder.

When you suffer from depression, you cannot face it alone. That is just the blunt truth. There are some of these depressions that only require an association to overcome them — for example, situational depression. Once you start feeling depressed, it is wise to speak out and let people help you before it grows into an incurable form of depression.

Depression can also be caused by some physical illnesses. The following are those illnesses that an individual can have and develop depression.

- Multiple sclerosis.

- Diabetes.

- Stroke.

- Alzheimer's disease.

- Parkinson's disease

- Epilepsy.

- Diabetes.

- Coronary heart disease.

- Rheumatoid arthritis.

- Systemic lupus erythematosus.

- HIV/AIDS.

If you know you are suffering from any of these types of illnesses, and you start noticing depressive disorder, it is advisable to visit your mental health practitioner.

Chapter five

THERAPIES THAT CAN HELP OVERCOME DEPRESSION

The following are three conventional therapies that have good records when it comes to treating depression.

Cognitive Behavioural Therapy (CBT)

Cognitive behavioural therapy is a type of psychotherapeutic treatment that helps patients understand the feelings and thoughts that influence behaviors. It helps penetrate and change negative thinking patterns associated with depression and handled by mental health counselors. CBT helps to be aware of negative thoughts so you can understand challenging problems clearly and respond to them effectively. It can be used to prevent a relapse of mental illness, discover ways you can manage emotions, cope with loss or grief, overcome depression or emotional trauma, treat mental illness when medications are not a good option, manage symptoms of psycho disease. The patient will learn coping strategies by recognizing negative thoughts.

Some of the mental health disorders that have improved as a result of Cognitive Behavioural Therapy (CBT) are;

- Depressive disorder

- Anxiety

- Eating disorder

- Bipolar disorder.

- Sexual disorder.

- Schizophrenia.

- Obsessive-compulsive disorder (OCD)

- Sleep disorder.

You can give it a try. It has been proven to have worked for a lot of people suffering from depression. It is an organised therapy that is limited to specified number of a visit that may be between 8 and 16 sessions.

Psychodynamic Therapy

This is primarily used to treat a patient suffering from depression and some other severe psychological disorders, most notably in the life of those who have lost meaning in their lives as a result of depression. It is also called insight-oriented therapy. The aim of this therapy is for self-awareness in the patient and understanding of the influence of the past and present behaviour. Because its theory is that feelings and harmful patterns are rooted in past experiences. During these sessions, the therapist tries to discover the root cause of the problem and then help change the psychology effect it has caused in the patient life.n it is goal-oriented and can take up to like 25 sessions. It is a long term therapy.

Interpersonal Therapy (IPT)

This is another method of treating depression. It is a type of psychotherapy that focuses on you and your relationships with other people. The therapist looks at personal relationships and encourages the patients to make some adjustments in life. The patient learns from the therapist on how to improve the problem, treat depression, and evaluate interactions to improve on how to relate with others. When a relationship with others is active, it reduces the tendencies of depressing moments. The techniques used during interpersonal therapy include;

- Identification of Emotions.

- Expression of emotion.

- You are dealing with emotional issues.

These three therapies have been tested, and they have been proven to be working. It has also helped solve or treat some depressive disorder in people.

Relating to your mental health practitioner

It is essential to regularly visit or talk to your doctor when you are depressed or taking an antidepressant, especially when you use any medication outside his consent. Also, as earlier mentioned, keep track of your symptoms and side effects you experience so that they can find the best remedy to tackle the type of depression.

 If you have a problem finding the right medication that can work for you, your doctor can use drug-genetic testing to determine the right option. If your depression is a result of pregnancy, become be sure to ask your doctor what medication is safest.

Some antidepressants carry cautions that they may increase suicidal thoughts, majorly among young people. It is advisable to let your doctor be aware if you are experiencing any suicidal thoughts to monitor your progress.

Above all, do not be discouraged if a particular medication, antidepressant, treatment, or therapy is not working for you. Be open enough to let your doctor be aware of what is wrong with you. With the information given in this book, be rest assure you will overcome depression.

Chapter six

HOW TO OVERCOME DEPRESSION BY LIFESTYLE

When you or your loved ones go through depression, it becomes challenging to gather that extra bit of strength to look after yourself. Slaying depression will come to effect when you take an active role in improving and steps that can help you battle depressive disorder. The following are some tested practices that can help you overcome depression alongside the counselling of medical practitioners.

- Engage yourself actively.

- Practice caring for yourself – engage in what makes you happy.

- Keep track of your low mood.

- Take good care of your body.

- Meet and connect with people

- Set targets for yourself.

- Avoid pretence

Engage yourself actively

When you engage yourself in active activities, this will also go a long way to helping you overcome depression. Take a step and join a group or forum.for example, the group may be a community project group, a sports team, or even a social media group or forum that can engage you in a discussion. The essence of this is to keep yourself engage with positivity so that you can close those little holes that allow mood swings. If eventually you are not elated by any of the old things you used to enjoy, leap of faith and find new ideas that can help you always get on your feet, such as volunteering. This will make you break out of unhelpful mood patterns and enhance your bright side.

Practice caring for yourself – engage in

what makes you happy.

As we grow, there is/are one or more things that will have discovered about ourselves, such as those things or activities either make you happy or unhappy. One of the ways to overcome depression is to figure out what works for you.

List those people, activities, and places that ignite the feel-good emotion in you. You can as well list your daily activities to figure out those once that ignite your happy-mood. It may be hard to include in the list all the things that make you happy, but try to incorporate the content elements, people, and places in your daily activities. For example, you might be the type that enjoys music, such as playing the piano, playing games or watching a movie. When this list is generated, ensure that you schedule time to observe them daily. By doing this, it is highly possible you overcome depression.

Keep track of your low mood

This question comes to you. How can I keep track of my depressed mood? It can be achieved by maintaining a mood diary. From the study, it has proved to help in keeping track of your changes in mood. This will help you sense the pattern of attitude that causes depression in you and enables you to work on it, know the right cure to use and also know what to tell your mental doctor. Additionally, when you keep track of your mood, you will know how to handle your day by not allowing your mood to dictate the outcome of your day.

Take good care of your body.

Quality sleep is vital when it comes to enhancing body functionality. Remember that depression can result from lack of sleep. Observing good sleep has been proved to show drastic improvement in people suffering from depression.

Another way of taking care of the body to overcome depression is to eat well – have a proper diet. A nutritious and healthy diet helps in enhancing physical and mental strength, and in turn, helps to increase your energy and improve your mood.

Additionally, improve with your hygiene such as taking a shower before you go out or dressing up well. This can act as a catalyst to brighten up your day.

As simple as these points mentioned above may seem, they have a positive effect on the outgrowing depression.

Meet and connect with people

A relationship is one of the strong tools to completely treat depression. Connect, meet, keep in touch, keep talking with people more than you used to. If, as a person meeting people physical is one of your weaknesses, there are several ways you can keep the bond of relationship stronger. You reach via phone calls, emails, text, and for faster response, you can use social media like facebook, facebook messenger, Whatsapp, and some other social media apps.

Try not to hide what you are going through. It is proven that many people have found comfort in sharing their experiences, and this act has helped a lot more overcome depression. Sometimes we feel our friends or family member will not understand. Your feelings may be wrong; why can't you try them. But if you think you won't be free discussing your problem with them, you can join a peer group support.you can as well join a group of people who face the same challenge, experiences, or have ones been in such a situation. From their skills and learning, you may eventually discover that you need to do to overcome your type of depression. And in like manner you will find joy seeing your skills have helped some people.

Set targets for yourself

You must ensure you are realistic when setting your goals or objectives. Setting unrealistic goals will mean disappointment when they are not met. The last thing you need to harbour is a negative feeling. Do not entertain negative emotions because they can trigger mood swings and eventually lead you to been depressed.

Set targets for yourself, so that you will be occupied in your mind. When you are working to achieve your goals, there will be little chances of having mood swings.

Avoid Pretence

Some people have escalated their depressive disorder by pretence. They shy away from treating themselves. This could mean taking long baths, spending quality time with your friends or your family. Do not forget to be kind to yourself. If you need your "me time," let nothing stop you from taking it.

These seven (7) will go a long way to help overcome depression or depressed state.

Chapter seven
MEDICAL WAY TO TREAT DEPRESSION

When depression in a patient has grown uncontrollably, different treatments are sorted to help manage the disorder. One of the treatments is the prescription of medicines. The medication prescribed is always an antidepressant.

When a patient suffering from depression is to be treated with medicine, the mental health practitioner begins with a low dose and subsequently increases the treatment if there is no improvement. The doctor monitors the improvement level of such a patient to know how the medicine works on him or her to avoid some severe side effects of the medications. For a start, the antidepressant may take up to four (4) to six (6) weeks to show any improvement in the patient.

Type of Medications to treat depression.

Medication is useful when it comes to treating the symptoms of depression. Antidepressant is medication a mental health practitioner will prescribe to you to tackle the problem of depression. But all antidepressants do not, however, work the same way. The antidepressant your doctor will prescribe to you is often base on your symptoms of depression, potential side effects, and some other factors. Most antidepressants work by stimulating chemicals in the brain. Those chemicals are known as neurotransmitters, and they include serotonin, norepinephrine, and dopamine, which are associated with depression. The class of antidepressants is determined by how the medication affects these neurotransmitters.

Monoamine oxidase inhibitors (MAOIs)

These are a class of drugs that inhibit the activity of one or both monoamine oxidase enzymes.they are best known as a powerful antidepressant, as well as an active therapeutic agent for panic disorder and social phobia. It works by ultimately effecting changes in the brain chemistry that are operational in depression. Examples of MAOIs drugs;

- Isocarboxazid (Marplan).
- Tranylcypromine (Parnate).
- Phenelzine (Nardi).

Monoamine oxidase inhibitors require a strict diet. Because of its interaction with foods such as cheese, wine, or pickles.

Atypical antidepressant

This is a type of antidepressant medication that acts in an atypical manner relative to most other antidepressants. It does not belong to any common category of antidepressants.in some cases they posses novel mechanism of action that are under development and in some cases they act faster than a typical antidepressant.

Example of atypical depressant.

- Trazodone vortioxetine (trintellix).

- Vilazodone (viibryd)

Atypical antipsychotic – second-generation Antipsychotic (SGA)

This category of medicines is used to treat a severe depressive disorder or used for Treatment-Resistant Depression (TRD). It is used to treat some particular mental or mood is order, which may include depression, which is our focus in this book and schizophrenia. Example of SGAs drugs are;

- Aripiprazole (Abilify)

- Quetiapine (Seroquel XR and Seroquel)

- Olanzapine (Zyprexa) is used with some other medications for effectiveness.

- Brexpiprazole (Rexulti); it helps to improve mood, appetite, sleep, and energy level and to treat schizophrenia.

Tricyclic antidepressants (TCAs)

These are antidepressants that have similar biological effects and chemical structure. It works similarly to serotonin and norepinephrine reuptake inhibitors (SNRI). Tricyclic antidepressants may be prescribed for patients that other drugs don't work for. Example of this antidepressants are;

- Nortriptyline (Pamelor).

- Imipramine (Tofranil).

- Doxepin.

- Desipramine (Norpramin).

- Amitriptyline.

Selective Serotonin Reuptake Inhibitors – SSRI

Serotonin is a monoamine neurotransmitter. It believed in contributing to the feelings of happiness and wellbeing. When you have a shortage of serotonin, it is believed you have a sad mood, negative thoughts, irritability, feeling tense, reduce interest in sex, low energy and much more. But our primary focus is on depression.

Selective serotonin reuptake inhibitors help relieve symptoms of depression by allowing the availability of serotonin. Examples of drugs that act as SSRIs are;

- Escitalopram (Lexapro)

- Sertraline (Zoloft).

- Citalopram (Celexa).

- Fluoxetine (Prozac)

There is a side effect of using this antidepressant. That is the reason the doctor monitors its impact on the patient.

Serotonin and Norepinephrine Reuptake Inhibitors – SNRI

Norepinephrine is a natural chemical in the body system that acts as a neurotransmitter and stress hormone – a substance that sends signals between the nerve cells. It is known to play an essential role in a person's mood and ability to concentrate. SNRI functions in a dual way by increasing the level of norepinephrine and serotonin that inhibit these substances that are absorbed back into the brain cells. Examples of SNRI drugs are;

- Levomilnacipran (fetzima)

- Venlafaxine (Effexor)

- Duloxetine (Cymbalta)

- Desvenlafaxine (Pristiq)

Norepinephrine-Dopamine Reuptake Inhibitors – NDRI

NDRIs helps to improve the concentration of mood regulators in the brain.it is used for clinical depression, narcolepsy, Attention deficit hyperactivity disorder (ADHD), and antiparkinson agents. Examples of norepinephrine-dopamine reuptake inhibitors include the following;

- Mirtazapine (Remeron).

- Bupropion (Wellbutrin, aplenzin, forfivo XL).

- Amineptine (survector, maneon).

- Difemetorex (cleofil).

- Ethylphenidate.

- Fencamfamine (glucoenergan, reactivan).

Newly approve antidepressant

There is some freshly approved antidepressants in the market. They include; selegiline (Emsam) and Ketamine nasal spray. It is also called spravato.

Chapter eight

OTHER TREATMENT THAT CAN BE USED

The following are other treatments you can use for someone suffering from depression.

Brain stimulation therapies

This can perform the role of treating some mental disorders. It involves activating the brain with electricity directly. This electricity can be through electrodes place in the scalp or directly implanted in the brain. Some of these brain stimulation therapies are mentioned below

- **Electroconvulsive Therapy (ECT):**

This is used to transmit short electrical impulses into the brain. It is used when treatment of severe depression such as (bipolar depression and schizophrenia) and treatment-resistance depression is required. This therapy is not just used for anybody suffering from depression, but for some patients that theirs as grown worse, maybe to committing suicide.

If para venture, you are approved for ECT. You will be anaesthetized to avoid pain, and you will be given muscle relaxants. During this process, the blood rate, heart rate, and breathing are monitored by the anesthesiologist. Electrodes are placed at the right points on the head, and an electric current passed through the brain. This causes a seizure that will last for at most one minute. This therapy may sound scary, but the patient won't feel the electrical impulses because he or she has been given a muscle relaxant and under anaesthesia. After the whole process, the patient is left to relax for a specific time. After at most ten minutes, the patient awakes, but after an hour, he or she is fit to resume his or her usual activities.

- **Repetitive Transcranial Magnetic stimulation (rTMS):**

This is another type of brain stimulation therapy that is similar to electroconvulsive Therapy ECT. The difference between both therapies is that ECT uses electric current while RTMS uses a magnet. It generates magnetic fields to stimulate nerve cells in the brain to improve symptoms of depression. Before the treatment, the doctor will determine the amount of magnetic energy required by the patient. This treatment lasts for forty minutes, and no anaesthesia is required.Also the patient remains awake during the process. Before the main treatment the patient would have passed through some series of tests and check-ups.

- **Deep Brain Stimulation (DBS):**

It is a surgery to implant a device that can send electrical signals to the brain. It was initially designed to reduce tremors from Parkinson's disease. The Food and Drug Administration FDA approves DBS to be used for the treatment of Obsessive-Compulsive Disorder. The use of DBS for the treatment of the depressive disorder is still under study. Likewise, its effectiveness and safety are not known for now.

- **Vagus Nerve Stimulation (VNS):**

This is used for the treatment of treatment-resistant disorder and major depressive disorder. It uses a pulse generator which is stationed at the upper side of the chest to stimulate the vagus nerve with electrical impulses. Vagus nerve sends messages to the part of the brain that controls sleep and mood. The FDA approved VNS to treat depression that has grown worse in a patient – Depression that does not show improvement after a lot of treatments and including the use of Electroconvulsive Therapy ECT. All the listed Brain stimulation therapies were given to open our eyes to possible treatment that can help treat depression. The decision is not for you to take after reading this book, but to have more understanding about how you can tackle your problem. Your mental health practitioner will know the best therapy that will be good for you, but you can as well ask questions on all these therapies. You never can tell, your curiosity may lead him to know the best treatment that should be given to you.

Lithium Treatment

Lithium has long been used for the treatment of the bipolar disorder. It is used as a mood stabilizer. It reduces the chances of suicidal action in a patient suffering from bipolar depression by sixty percent (60%). Lithium serves as an anti-manic agent. It is used to prevent or treat phase of Mania in people suffering from bipolar depression or manic depressive disorder.

Majorly for the treatment of bipolar depression, lithium therapy is the most widely used therapy. Lithium works best if the amount of drugs in your body system is kept at uniform level. It hinders the flow of sodium through the nerve or muscle cells in the body and sodium prevents excitation.

Mood stabilizers like lithium are manufactured to treat bipolar depression or related depressive disorder. When using these drugs for treatment, you must strictly adhere to the instruction of your mental practitioner to avoid overdose or abuse. This is because of anybody that abuse the use of these drugs should know that lithium does not only result in high but also a toxic side effect when abusively used.

Thyroid treatment

When using thyroid treatment for someone suffering from depression, maybe unipolar depression, thyroid hormone can serve as two different functions.

1. As augmentation for a patient whose response to antidepressant monotherapy is low.

2. It can also be used to accelerate response in a patient when compared with tricyclic antidepressant monotherapy.this is because thyroid hormones can work simultaneously with tricyclic at the start of pharmacotherapy.

Psychedelics Treatment

This type of treatment is still on study. When a depressed patient is being treated with this therapy, he/ she is thoroughly monitored for better results. Psychedelics are the psychoactive ingredients in mushroom, which may include LSD and psilocybin.

About the Author

ADEGBOYE SAMUEL is an author, public speaker parenting expert, and author. He has spent much of his life, rendering help to get people out of depression through counseling, his publications, and as an author.

Samuel is aware of the challenges faced by people suffering from this illness. With his innovative and powerful approach to help victims achieve their goals, Samuel aims at redefining the methods generally used for the treatment of depression and he was able to treat a lot of patients in the past years successfully.

Samuel is a mentor and consultant, for teens, young ones and adult to help them overcome their fears, have a fruitful relationship, and lead happier lives.

Acknowledgements

First of all, my appreciation goes to God, Almighty, for the opportunity to collate this manuscript. I am grateful for several friends, colleagues, and co-members in encouraging and supporting me to start the work, persevere with it, and finally to publish it.

THANKS FOR READING

www.ingramcontent.com/pod-product-compliance
Lightning Source LLC
Chambersburg PA
CBHW052119030426
42335CB00025B/3055